FORWORD

Here we go. You want to change bad habits? You finally want to be regularly active and get your fit on? Then you've bought just the right book with this 90 Days new me Journal.

This book gives you a training plan for the next 90 days. This way you will build not only momentum to keep going, but new habits that will change you.

A few important points:

1. Maybe you don't know every exercise yet, thats ok. Exercises and training days will be repeated until you are **moving like a pro**.

2. If you don't know an exercise, just enter the name on **YouTube**, You'll find instructions on how to do each exercise.

3. If you feel that you can't do the full training for the day, **slow down** and try to do as much as you can. But always remember: **Health comes first.**

4. Even if you have to skip a training day because you're sick or just can't make it, **don't worry**. Just continue with the next training.

5. Try to develop **healthy habits**. Here are a few examples:
   a. Take the stairs, not the elevator.
   b. Eat less processed food.
   c. More veggies and fruit.
   d. Try to walk more, don't always take the car.
   e. Water Water Water (drink it, of course.)
   f. Try to average 7-8h of sleep each night.
   g. Enjoy the Ride!

And now it's **GAMETIME!**
Off to the fittest **90 days** of your life!

HOW TO USE THIS JOURNAL

Write down everything you eat: Breakfast, Lunch, Dinner and Snacks

Track your water intake. One Glass = 0,5 Liters.

DAY 1

BREAKFAST

DINNER

LUNCH

SNACK

TODAYS WATER INTAKE

TODAYS SLEEP

SLEEP QUALITY

0   10

I HAVE SLEPT ..... HOURS

TODAYS FEELINGS

WORKOUT OF THE DAY

☐ 100 JUMPING JACKS

☐ 70 RUSSIAN TWISTS

☐ 50 CRUNCHES

☐ 20 STANDING CALF RAISES

☐ 20 TRICEP DIPS

☐ PUSH-UPS

☐ 5 SQUATS

☐ 30 SECONDS PLANK

☐ 20 LUNGES (EACH SIDE)

☐ LUNGE SPLIT JUMPS

How did you sleep? Rate from 1 - 10. 1 Being horrible and 10 heavenlike. Also how many hours did you sleep?

Your Workout of the day!

How do you feel today? 1 Star = Like S**T - 3 Star = Bring it on!

CROSS A BIG X OVER EVERY DAY YOU'VE ROCKED!

This way you will see what you already have accomplished and what lays ahead. Get motivated, prepared and build

MOMENTUM

1	2	3	4	5	6	7	8	9	10
11	12	13	14	15	16	17	18	19	20
21	22	23	24	25	26	27	28	29	30
31	32	33	34	35	36	37	38	39	40
41	42	43	44	45	46	47	48	49	50
51	52	53	54	55	56	57	58	59	60
61	62	63	64	65	66	67	68	69	70
71	72	73	74	75	76	77	78	79	80
81	82	83	84	85	86	87	88	89	90

DAY 1

BREAKFAST

....
....
....
....

LUNCH

....
....
....
....

DINNER

....
....
....
....

SNACK

....
....
....
....

TODAYS WATER INTAKE

TODAYS SLEEP

SLEEP QUALITY

| 0 | 5 | 10 |

I HAVE SLEPT ..... HOURS

TODAYS FEELINGS

WORKOUT OF THE DAY

- ☐ 100 JUMPING JACKS
- ☐ 50 CRUNCHES
- ☐ 20 TRICEP DIPS
- ☐ 15 SQUATS
- ☐ 20 LUNGES (EACH SIDE)
- ☐ 70 RUSSIAN TWISTS
- ☐ 20 STANDING CALF RAISES
- ☐ 5 PUSH-UPS
- ☐ 30 SECONDS PLANK
- ☐ 10 LUNGE SPLIT JUMPS

DAY 2

BREAKFAST
....
....
....
....

LUNCH
....
....
....
....

DINNER
....
....
....
....

SNACK
....
....
....

TODAYS WATER INTAKE

TODAYS SLEEP

SLEEP QUALITY

0   5   10

I HAVE SLEPT ..... HOURS

TODAYS FEELINGS

☆ ☆ ☆

WORKOUT OF THE DAY

- ☐ 80 JUMPING JACKS
- ☐ 50 VERTICAL LEG CRUNCHES
- ☐ 20 SIT-UPS
- ☐ 15 TRICEP DIPS
- ☐ 20 SQUATS
- ☐ 10 SIDE LUNGES (EACH LEG)
- ☐ 15 LEG LIFTS (EACH LEG)
- ☐ 50 BICYCLES
- ☐ 15 WALL PUSH-UPS
- ☐ 40 RUSSIAN TWISTS

DAY 3

BREAKFAST

....
....
....
....

LUNCH

....
....
....
....

DINNER

....
....
....
....

SNACK

....
....
....
....

TODAYS WATER INTAKE

TODAYS SLEEP

SLEEP QUALITY

0   5   10

I HAVE SLEPT ..... HOURS

TODAYS FEELINGS

WORKOUT OF THE DAY

- ☐ 90 JUMPING JACKS
- ☐ 20 TRICEP DIPS
- ☐ 10 SIT-UPS
- ☐ 30 SECONDS PLANK
- ☐ 30 SQUATS
- ☐ 15 INCLINE PUSH-UPS
- ☐ 40 CRUNCHES
- ☐ 10 OBLIQUE CRUNCHES (EACH SIDE)
- ☐ 20 STANDING CALF RAISES

DAY 4

BREAKFAST

....

....

....

....

LUNCH

....

....

....

....

DINNER

....

....

....

....

SNACK

....

....

....

TODAYS WATER INTAKE

TODAYS SLEEP

SLEEP QUALITY

0   5   10

I HAVE SLEPT ..... HOURS

TODAYS FEELINGS

☆ ☆ ☆

WORKOUT OF THE DAY

☐ 100 JUMPING JACKS

☐ 25 VERTICAL LEG CRUNCHES

☐ 30 CRUNCHES

☐ 20 SQUATS

☐ 20 WALL PUSH-UPS

☐ 50 RUSSIAN TWISTS

☐ 15 SECONDS SIDE PLANK (EACH SIDE)

☐ 10 LUNGE SPLIT JUMPS

☐ 5 JUMP SQUATS

☐ 40 HIGH KNEES

DAY 5

BREAKFAST

....
....
....
....

LUNCH

....
....
....
....

DINNER

....
....
....
....

SNACK

....
....
....
....

TODAYS WATER INTAKE

TODAYS SLEEP

SLEEP QUALITY

0   5   10

I HAVE SLEPT ..... HOURS

TODAYS FEELINGS

WORKOUT OF THE DAY

- [ ] 60 JUMPING JACKS
- [ ] 40 CRUNCHES
- [ ] 10 SIT-UPS
- [ ] 10 TRICEP DIPS
- [ ] 20 SIDE LUNGES (EACH SIDE)

- [ ] 15 INCLINE PUSH-UPS
- [ ] 10 OBLIQUE CRUNCHES (EACH SIDE)
- [ ] 30 BUTT KICKERS
- [ ] 5 JUMP SQUATS
- [ ] 10 JACK KNIFE SIT-UPS

DAY 6

BREAKFAST

....
....
....
....

LUNCH

....
....
....
....

DINNER

....
....
....
....

SNACK

....
....
....
....

TODAYS WATER INTAKE

TODAYS SLEEP

SLEEP QUALITY

0   5   10

I HAVE SLEPT ..... HOURS

TODAYS FEELINGS

WORKOUT OF THE DAY

- ☐ 50 JUMPING JACKS
- ☐ 20 SQUATS
- ☐ 100 RUSSIAN TWISTS
- ☐ 5 KNEELING PUSH-UPS
- ☐ 1 MINUTE DOWNWARD DOG
- ☐ 15 JACK KNIFE SIT-UPS
- ☐ 10 LUNGES (EACH SIDE)
- ☐ 10 SIDE LUNGES (EACH SIDE)
- ☐ 20 INNER THIGH LIFTS (EACH SIDE)

DAY 7

BREAKFAST

....

....

....

....

LUNCH

....

....

....

....

DINNER

....

....

....

....

SNACK

....

....

....

....

TODAYS WATER INTAKE

TODAYS SLEEP

SLEEP QUALITY

0   5   10

I HAVE SLEPT ..... HOURS

TODAYS FEELINGS

☆ ☆ ☆

WORKOUT OF THE DAY

☐ 45 JUMPING JACKS

☐ 15 SQUATS

☐ 5 JUMP SQUATS

☐ 50 RUSSIAN TWISTS

☐ 30 SECONDS PLANK

☐ 10 STANDING CALF RAISES

☐ 5 KNEELING PUSH-UPS

☐ 30 SECONDS SUPERMAN

☐ 10 LUNGES (EACH SIDE)

☐ 40 CRUNCHES

DAY 8

BREAKFAST
....
....
....
....

DINNER
....
....
....

LUNCH
....
....
....
....

SNACK
....
....
....

TODAYS WATER INTAKE

TODAYS SLEEP

SLEEP QUALITY

0   5   10

I HAVE SLEPT ..... HOURS

TODAYS FEELINGS

WORKOUT OF THE DAY

- ☐ 100 JUMPING JACKS
- ☐ 50 CRUNCHES
- ☐ 20 TRICEP DIPS
- ☐ 15 SQUATS
- ☐ 20 LUNGES (EACH SIDE)
- ☐ 70 RUSSIAN TWISTS
- ☐ 20 STANDING CALF RAISES
- ☐ 5 PUSH-UPS
- ☐ 30 SECONDS PLANK
- ☐ 10 LUNGE SPLIT JUMPS

DAY 9

BREAKFAST

....
....
....
....

LUNCH

....
....
....
....

DINNER

....
....
....
....

SNACK

....
....
....
....

TODAYS WATER INTAKE

TODAYS SLEEP

SLEEP QUALITY

0   5   10

I HAVE SLEPT ..... HOURS

TODAYS FEELINGS

WORKOUT OF THE DAY

- ☐ 80 JUMPING JACKS
- ☐ 50 VERTICAL LEG CRUNCHES
- ☐ 20 SIT-UPS
- ☐ 15 TRICEP DIPS
- ☐ 20 SQUATS
- ☐ 10 SIDE LUNGES (EACH LEG)
- ☐ 15 LEG LIFTS (EACH LEG)
- ☐ 50 BICYCLES
- ☐ 15 WALL PUSH-UPS
- ☐ 40 RUSSIAN TWISTS

DAY 10

BREAKFAST

....

....

....

....

LUNCH

....

....

....

....

DINNER

....

....

....

....

SNACK

....

....

....

....

TODAYS WATER INTAKE

TODAYS SLEEP

SLEEP QUALITY

0   5   10

I HAVE SLEPT ..... HOURS

TODAYS FEELINGS

WORKOUT OF THE DAY

- ☐ 90 JUMPING JACKS
- ☐ 20 TRICEP DIPS
- ☐ 10 SIT-UPS
- ☐ 30 SECONDS PLANK
- ☐ 30 SQUATS
- ☐ 15 INCLINE PUSH-UPS
- ☐ 40 CRUNCHES
- ☐ 10 OBLIQUE CRUNCHES (EACH SIDE)
- ☐ 20 STANDING CALF RAISES

DAY 11

BREAKFAST

....
....
....
....

LUNCH

....
....
....
....

DINNER

....
....
....

SNACK

....
....
....

TODAYS WATER INTAKE

TODAYS SLEEP

SLEEP QUALITY

0   5   10

I HAVE SLEPT ..... HOURS

TODAYS FEELINGS

WORKOUT OF THE DAY

- ☐ 100 JUMPING JACKS
- ☐ 25 VERTICAL LEG CRUNCHES
- ☐ 30 CRUNCHES
- ☐ 20 SQUATS
- ☐ 20 WALL PUSH–UPS
- ☐ 50 RUSSIAN TWISTS
- ☐ 15 SECONDS SIDE PLANK (EACH SIDE)
- ☐ 10 LUNGE SPLIT JUMPS
- ☐ 5 JUMP SQUATS
- ☐ 40 HIGH KNEES

DAY 12

BREAKFAST

....
....
....
....

LUNCH

....
....
....
....

DINNER

....
....
....
....

SNACK

....
....
....
....

TODAYS WATER INTAKE

TODAYS SLEEP

SLEEP QUALITY

| 0 | 5 | 10 |

I HAVE SLEPT ..... HOURS

TODAYS FEELINGS

☆ ☆ ☆

WORKOUT OF THE DAY

☐ 60 JUMPING JACKS

☐ 40 CRUNCHES

☐ 10 SIT-UPS

☐ 10 TRICEP DIPS

☐ 20 SIDE LUNGES (EACH SIDE)

☐ 15 INCLINE PUSH-UPS

☐ 10 OBLIQUE CRUNCHES (EACH SIDE)

☐ 30 BUTT KICKERS

☐ 5 JUMP SQUATS

☐ 10 JACK KNIFE SIT-UPS

DAY 13

BREAKFAST

....
....
....
....

LUNCH

....
....
....
....

DINNER

....
....
....
....

SNACK

....
....
....
....

TODAYS WATER INTAKE

TODAYS SLEEP

SLEEP QUALITY

0   5   10

I HAVE SLEPT ..... HOURS

TODAYS FEELINGS

WORKOUT OF THE DAY

☐ 50 JUMPING JACKS

☐ 20 SQUATS

☐ 100 RUSSIAN TWISTS

☐ 5 KNEELING PUSH-UPS

☐ 1 MINUTE DOWNWARD DOG

☐ 15 JACK KNIFE SIT-UPS

☐ 10 LUNGES (EACH SIDE)

☐ 10 SIDE LUNGES (EACH SIDE)

☐ 20 INNER THIGH LIFTS (EACH SIDE)

DAY 14

BREAKFAST

....

....

....

....

LUNCH

....

....

....

....

DINNER

....

....

....

....

SNACK

....

....

....

....

TODAYS WATER INTAKE

TODAYS SLEEP

SLEEP QUALITY

| 0 | 5 | 10 |

I HAVE SLEPT ..... HOURS

TODAYS FEELINGS

☆ ☆ ☆

WORKOUT OF THE DAY

☐ 45 JUMPING JACKS

☐ 15 SQUATS

☐ 5 JUMP SQUATS

☐ 50 RUSSIAN TWISTS

☐ 30 SECONDS PLANK

☐ 10 STANDING CALF RAISES

☐ 5 KNEELING PUSH-UPS

☐ 30 SECONDS SUPERMAN

☐ 10 LUNGES (EACH SIDE)

☐ 40 CRUNCHES

DAY 15

BREAKFAST

....
....
....
....

LUNCH

....
....
....
....

DINNER

....
....
....
....

SNACK

....
....
....
....

TODAYS WATER INTAKE

TODAYS SLEEP

SLEEP QUALITY

0   5   10

I HAVE SLEPT ..... HOURS

TODAYS FEELINGS

WORKOUT OF THE DAY

- ☐ 100 JUMPING JACKS
- ☐ 50 CRUNCHES
- ☐ 20 TRICEP DIPS
- ☐ 15 SQUATS
- ☐ 20 LUNGES (EACH SIDE)
- ☐ 70 RUSSIAN TWISTS
- ☐ 20 STANDING CALF RAISES
- ☐ 5 PUSH-UPS
- ☐ 30 SECONDS PLANK
- ☐ 10 LUNGE SPLIT JUMPS

DAY 16

BREAKFAST
....
....
....
....

LUNCH
....
....
....
....

DINNER
....
....
....
....

SNACK
....
....
....
....

TODAYS WATER INTAKE

TODAYS SLEEP

SLEEP QUALITY

| 0 | 5 | 10 |

I HAVE SLEPT ..... HOURS

TODAYS FEELINGS

☆ ☆ ☆

WORKOUT OF THE DAY

☐ 80 JUMPING JACKS

☐ 50 VERTICAL LEG CRUNCHES

☐ 20 SIT-UPS

☐ 15 TRICEP DIPS

☐ 20 SQUATS

☐ 10 SIDE LUNGES (EACH LEG)

☐ 15 LEG LIFTS (EACH LEG)

☐ 50 BICYCLES

☐ 15 WALL PUSH-UPS

☐ 40 RUSSIAN TWISTS

DAY 17

BREAKFAST

....
....
....
....

LUNCH

....
....
....
....

DINNER

....
....
....
....

SNACK

....
....
....
....

TODAYS WATER INTAKE

TODAYS SLEEP

SLEEP QUALITY

0   5   10

I HAVE SLEPT ..... HOURS

TODAYS FEELINGS

☆ ☆ ☆

WORKOUT OF THE DAY

- ☐ 90 JUMPING JACKS
- ☐ 20 TRICEP DIPS
- ☐ 10 SIT-UPS
- ☐ 30 SECONDS PLANK
- ☐ 30 SQUATS
- ☐ 15 INCLINE PUSH-UPS
- ☐ 40 CRUNCHES
- ☐ 10 OBLIQUE CRUNCHES (EACH SIDE)
- ☐ 20 STANDING CALF RAISES

DAY 18

BREAKFAST

....
....
....
....

LUNCH

....
....
....
....

DINNER

....
....
....
....

SNACK

....
....
....
....

TODAYS WATER INTAKE

TODAYS SLEEP

SLEEP QUALITY

0   5   10

I HAVE SLEPT ..... HOURS

TODAYS FEELINGS

WORKOUT OF THE DAY

- ☐ 100 JUMPING JACKS
- ☐ 25 VERTICAL LEG CRUNCHES
- ☐ 30 CRUNCHES
- ☐ 20 SQUATS
- ☐ 20 WALL PUSH-UPS
- ☐ 50 RUSSIAN TWISTS
- ☐ 15 SECONDS SIDE PLANK (EACH SIDE)
- ☐ 10 LUNGE SPLIT JUMPS
- ☐ 5 JUMP SQUATS
- ☐ 40 HIGH KNEES

DAY 19

BREAKFAST

....
....
....
....

LUNCH

....
....
....
....

DINNER

....
....
....

SNACK

....
....
....
....

TODAYS WATER INTAKE

TODAYS SLEEP

SLEEP QUALITY

0   5   10

I HAVE SLEPT ..... HOURS

TODAYS FEELINGS

WORKOUT OF THE DAY

- ☐ 60 JUMPING JACKS
- ☐ 40 CRUNCHES
- ☐ 10 SIT-UPS
- ☐ 10 TRICEP DIPS
- ☐ 20 SIDE LUNGES (EACH SIDE)
- ☐ 15 INCLINE PUSH-UPS
- ☐ 10 OBLIQUE CRUNCHES (EACH SIDE)
- ☐ 30 BUTT KICKERS
- ☐ 5 JUMP SQUATS
- ☐ 10 JACK KNIFE SIT-UPS

DAY 20

BREAKFAST

....
....
....
....

LUNCH

....
....
....
....

DINNER

....
....
....
....

SNACK

....
....
....
....

TODAYS WATER INTAKE

TODAYS SLEEP

SLEEP QUALITY

```
0            5            10
```

I HAVE SLEPT ..... HOURS

TODAYS FEELINGS

WORKOUT OF THE DAY

- ☐ 50 JUMPING JACKS
- ☐ 20 SQUATS
- ☐ 100 RUSSIAN TWISTS
- ☐ 5 KNEELING PUSH-UPS
- ☐ 1 MINUTE DOWNWARD DOG
- ☐ 15 JACK KNIFE SIT-UPS
- ☐ 10 LUNGES (EACH SIDE)
- ☐ 10 SIDE LUNGES (EACH SIDE)
- ☐ 20 INNER THIGH LIFTS (EACH SIDE)

DAY 21

BREAKFAST

....
....
....
....

LUNCH

....
....
....
....

DINNER

....
....
....
....

SNACK

....
....
....
....

TODAYS WATER INTAKE

TODAYS SLEEP

SLEEP QUALITY

0   5   10

I HAVE SLEPT ..... HOURS

TODAYS FEELINGS

WORKOUT OF THE DAY

- ☐ 45 JUMPING JACKS
- ☐ 15 SQUATS
- ☐ 5 JUMP SQUATS
- ☐ 50 RUSSIAN TWISTS
- ☐ 30 SECONDS PLANK
- ☐ 10 STANDING CALF RAISES
- ☐ 5 KNEELING PUSH-UPS
- ☐ 30 SECONDS SUPERMAN
- ☐ 10 LUNGES (EACH SIDE)
- ☐ 40 CRUNCHES

DAY 22

BREAKFAST

....
....
....
....

LUNCH

....
....
....
....

DINNER

....
....
....
....

SNACK

....
....
....
....

TODAYS WATER INTAKE

TODAYS SLEEP

SLEEP QUALITY

| 0 | 5 | 10 |

I HAVE SLEPT ..... HOURS

TODAYS FEELINGS

☆ ☆ ☆

WORKOUT OF THE DAY

- ☐ 100 JUMPING JACKS
- ☐ 50 CRUNCHES
- ☐ 20 TRICEP DIPS
- ☐ 15 SQUATS
- ☐ 20 LUNGES (EACH SIDE)
- ☐ 70 RUSSIAN TWISTS
- ☐ 20 STANDING CALF RAISES
- ☐ 5 PUSH-UPS
- ☐ 30 SECONDS PLANK
- ☐ 10 LUNGE SPLIT JUMPS

DAY 23

BREAKFAST

....
....
....
....

DINNER

....
....
....
....

LUNCH

....
....
....
....

SNACK

....
....
....
....

TODAYS WATER INTAKE

TODAYS SLEEP

SLEEP QUALITY

0   5   10

I HAVE SLEPT ..... HOURS

TODAYS FEELINGS

☆ ☆ ☆

WORKOUT OF THE DAY

- ☐ 80 JUMPING JACKS
- ☐ 50 VERTICAL LEG CRUNCHES
- ☐ 20 SIT-UPS
- ☐ 15 TRICEP DIPS
- ☐ 20 SQUATS
- ☐ 10 SIDE LUNGES (EACH LEG)
- ☐ 15 LEG LIFTS (EACH LEG)
- ☐ 50 BICYCLES
- ☐ 15 WALL PUSH-UPS
- ☐ 40 RUSSIAN TWISTS

DAY 24

BREAKFAST

....

....

....

....

LUNCH

....

....

....

....

DINNER

....

....

....

....

SNACK

....

....

....

....

TODAYS WATER INTAKE

TODAYS SLEEP

SLEEP QUALITY

0   5   10

I HAVE SLEPT ..... HOURS

TODAYS FEELINGS

☆ ☆ ☆

WORKOUT OF THE DAY

☐ 90 JUMPING JACKS

☐ 20 TRICEP DIPS

☐ 10 SIT-UPS

☐ 30 SECONDS PLANK

☐ 30 SQUATS

☐ 15 INCLINE PUSH-UPS

☐ 40 CRUNCHES

☐ 10 OBLIQUE CRUNCHES (EACH SIDE)

☐ 20 STANDING CALF RAISES

DAY 25

BREAKFAST

....
....
....
....

LUNCH

....
....
....
....

DINNER

....
....
....
....

SNACK

....
....
....
....

TODAYS WATER INTAKE

TODAYS SLEEP

SLEEP QUALITY

0   5   10

I HAVE SLEPT ..... HOURS

TODAYS FEELINGS

☆ ☆ ☆

WORKOUT OF THE DAY

☐ 100 JUMPING JACKS

☐ 25 VERTICAL LEG CRUNCHES

☐ 30 CRUNCHES

☐ 20 SQUATS

☐ 20 WALL PUSH-UPS

☐ 50 RUSSIAN TWISTS

☐ 15 SECONDS SIDE PLANK (EACH SIDE)

☐ 10 LUNGE SPLIT JUMPS

☐ 5 JUMP SQUATS

☐ 40 HIGH KNEES

DAY 26

BREAKFAST

....
....
....
....

LUNCH

....
....
....
....

DINNER

....
....
....

SNACK

....
....
....
....

TODAYS WATER INTAKE

TODAYS SLEEP

SLEEP QUALITY

| 0 | 5 | 10 |

I HAVE SLEPT ..... HOURS

TODAYS FEELINGS

☆ ☆ ☆

WORKOUT OF THE DAY

- ☐ 60 JUMPING JACKS
- ☐ 40 CRUNCHES
- ☐ 10 SIT-UPS
- ☐ 10 TRICEP DIPS
- ☐ 20 SIDE LUNGES (EACH SIDE)
- ☐ 15 INCLINE PUSH-UPS
- ☐ 10 OBLIQUE CRUNCHES (EACH SIDE)
- ☐ 30 BUTT KICKERS
- ☐ 5 JUMP SQUATS
- ☐ 10 JACK KNIFE SIT-UPS

DAY 27

BREAKFAST

....
....
....
....

LUNCH

....
....
....
....

DINNER

....
....
....
....

SNACK

....
....
....
....

TODAYS WATER INTAKE

TODAYS SLEEP

SLEEP QUALITY

0   5   10

I HAVE SLEPT ..... HOURS

TODAYS FEELINGS

WORKOUT OF THE DAY

- [ ] 50 JUMPING JACKS
- [ ] 20 SQUATS
- [ ] 100 RUSSIAN TWISTS
- [ ] 5 KNEELING PUSH-UPS
- [ ] 1 MINUTE DOWNWARD DOG
- [ ] 15 JACK KNIFE SIT-UPS
- [ ] 10 LUNGES (EACH SIDE)
- [ ] 10 SIDE LUNGES (EACH SIDE)
- [ ] 20 INNER THIGH LIFTS (EACH SIDE)

DAY 28

BREAKFAST

....
....
....
....

LUNCH

....
....
....
....

DINNER

....
....
....
....

SNACK

....
....
....
....

TODAYS WATER INTAKE

TODAYS SLEEP

SLEEP QUALITY

0   5   10

I HAVE SLEPT ..... HOURS

TODAYS FEELINGS

☆ ☆ ☆

WORKOUT OF THE DAY

☐ 45 JUMPING JACKS

☐ 15 SQUATS

☐ 5 JUMP SQUATS

☐ 50 RUSSIAN TWISTS

☐ 30 SECONDS PLANK

☐ 10 STANDING CALF RAISES

☐ 5 KNEELING PUSH-UPS

☐ 30 SECONDS SUPERMAN

☐ 10 LUNGES (EACH SIDE)

☐ 40 CRUNCHES

DAY 29

BREAKFAST

....

....

....

....

LUNCH

....

....

....

....

DINNER

....

....

....

....

SNACK

....

....

....

....

TODAYS WATER INTAKE

TODAYS SLEEP

SLEEP QUALITY

| 0 | 5 | 10 |

I HAVE SLEPT ..... HOURS

TODAYS FEELINGS

☆ ☆ ☆

WORKOUT OF THE DAY

☐ 100 JUMPING JACKS

☐ 50 CRUNCHES

☐ 20 TRICEP DIPS

☐ 15 SQUATS

☐ 20 LUNGES (EACH SIDE)

☐ 70 RUSSIAN TWISTS

☐ 20 STANDING CALF RAISES

☐ 5 PUSH-UPS

☐ 30 SECONDS PLANK

☐ 10 LUNGE SPLIT JUMPS

DAY 30

BREAKFAST

....
....
....
....

LUNCH

....
....
....
....

DINNER

....
....
....
....

SNACK

....
....
....

TODAYS WATER INTAKE

TODAYS SLEEP

SLEEP QUALITY

0   5   10

I HAVE SLEPT ..... HOURS

TODAYS FEELINGS

☆ ☆ ☆

WORKOUT OF THE DAY

☐ 80 JUMPING JACKS

☐ 50 VERTICAL LEG CRUNCHES

☐ 20 SIT-UPS

☐ 15 TRICEP DIPS

☐ 20 SQUATS

☐ 10 SIDE LUNGES (EACH LEG)

☐ 15 LEG LIFTS (EACH LEG)

☐ 50 BICYCLES

☐ 15 WALL PUSH-UPS

☐ 40 RUSSIAN TWISTS

DAY 31

BREAKFAST

....
....
....
....

LUNCH

....
....
....
....

DINNER

....
....
....
....

SNACK

....
....
....
....

TODAYS WATER INTAKE

TODAYS SLEEP

SLEEP QUALITY

0   5   10

I HAVE SLEPT ..... HOURS

TODAYS FEELINGS

WORKOUT OF THE DAY

- ☐ 90 JUMPING JACKS
- ☐ 20 TRICEP DIPS
- ☐ 10 SIT-UPS
- ☐ 30 SECONDS PLANK
- ☐ 30 SQUATS
- ☐ 15 INCLINE PUSH-UPS
- ☐ 40 CRUNCHES
- ☐ 10 OBLIQUE CRUNCHES (EACH SIDE)
- ☐ 20 STANDING CALF RAISES

DAY 32

BREAKFAST

....
....
....
....

LUNCH

....
....
....
....

DINNER

....
....
....

SNACK

....
....
....
....

TODAYS WATER INTAKE

TODAYS SLEEP

SLEEP QUALITY

| 0 | 5 | 10 |

I HAVE SLEPT ..... HOURS

TODAYS FEELINGS

WORKOUT OF THE DAY

- ☐ 100 JUMPING JACKS
- ☐ 25 VERTICAL LEG CRUNCHES
- ☐ 30 CRUNCHES
- ☐ 20 SQUATS
- ☐ 20 WALL PUSH-UPS
- ☐ 50 RUSSIAN TWISTS
- ☐ 15 SECONDS SIDE PLANK (EACH SIDE)
- ☐ 10 LUNGE SPLIT JUMPS
- ☐ 5 JUMP SQUATS
- ☐ 40 HIGH KNEES

DAY 33

BREAKFAST

....

....

....

....

LUNCH

....

....

....

....

DINNER

....

....

....

....

SNACK

....

....

....

....

TODAYS WATER INTAKE

TODAYS SLEEP

SLEEP QUALITY

0   5   10

I HAVE SLEPT ..... HOURS

TODAYS FEELINGS

WORKOUT OF THE DAY

- ☐ 60 JUMPING JACKS
- ☐ 40 CRUNCHES
- ☐ 10 SIT-UPS
- ☐ 10 TRICEP DIPS
- ☐ 20 SIDE LUNGES (EACH SIDE)
- ☐ 15 INCLINE PUSH-UPS
- ☐ 10 OBLIQUE CRUNCHES (EACH SIDE)
- ☐ 30 BUTT KICKERS
- ☐ 5 JUMP SQUATS
- ☐ 10 JACK KNIFE SIT-UPS

DAY 34

BREAKFAST

....
....
....
....

LUNCH

....
....
....
....

DINNER

....
....
....
....

SNACK

....
....
....
....

TODAYS WATER INTAKE

TODAYS SLEEP

SLEEP QUALITY

| 0 | 5 | 10 |

I HAVE SLEPT ..... HOURS

TODAYS FEELINGS

WORKOUT OF THE DAY

- ☐ 50 JUMPING JACKS
- ☐ 20 SQUATS
- ☐ 100 RUSSIAN TWISTS
- ☐ 5 KNEELING PUSH-UPS
- ☐ 1 MINUTE DOWNWARD DOG
- ☐ 15 JACK KNIFE SIT-UPS
- ☐ 10 LUNGES (EACH SIDE)
- ☐ 10 SIDE LUNGES (EACH SIDE)
- ☐ 20 INNER THIGH LIFTS (EACH SIDE)

DAY 35

BREAKFAST

....

....

....

....

LUNCH

....

....

....

....

DINNER

....

....

....

....

SNACK

....

....

....

....

TODAYS WATER INTAKE

TODAYS SLEEP

SLEEP QUALITY

0   5   10

I HAVE SLEPT ..... HOURS

TODAYS FEELINGS

WORKOUT OF THE DAY

- [ ] 45 JUMPING JACKS
- [ ] 15 SQUATS
- [ ] 5 JUMP SQUATS
- [ ] 50 RUSSIAN TWISTS
- [ ] 30 SECONDS PLANK
- [ ] 10 STANDING CALF RAISES
- [ ] 5 KNEELING PUSH-UPS
- [ ] 30 SECONDS SUPERMAN
- [ ] 10 LUNGES (EACH SIDE)
- [ ] 40 CRUNCHES

DAY 36

BREAKFAST
....
....
....

LUNCH
....
....
....
....

DINNER
....
....
....
....

SNACK
....
....
....
....

TODAYS WATER INTAKE

TODAYS SLEEP

SLEEP QUALITY

| 0 | 5 | 10 |

I HAVE SLEPT ..... HOURS

TODAYS FEELINGS

WORKOUT OF THE DAY

- ☐ 100 JUMPING JACKS
- ☐ 50 CRUNCHES
- ☐ 20 TRICEP DIPS
- ☐ 15 SQUATS
- ☐ 20 LUNGES (EACH SIDE)
- ☐ 70 RUSSIAN TWISTS
- ☐ 20 STANDING CALF RAISES
- ☐ 5 PUSH-UPS
- ☐ 30 SECONDS PLANK
- ☐ 10 LUNGE SPLIT JUMPS

DAY 37

BREAKFAST

....
....
....
....

LUNCH

....
....
....
....

DINNER

....
....
....
....

SNACK

....
....
....
....

TODAYS WATER INTAKE

TODAYS SLEEP

SLEEP QUALITY

0	5	10

I HAVE SLEPT ..... HOURS

TODAYS FEELINGS

☆ ☆ ☆

WORKOUT OF THE DAY

- ☐ 80 JUMPING JACKS
- ☐ 50 VERTICAL LEG CRUNCHES
- ☐ 20 SIT-UPS
- ☐ 15 TRICEP DIPS
- ☐ 20 SQUATS
- ☐ 10 SIDE LUNGES (EACH LEG)
- ☐ 15 LEG LIFTS (EACH LEG)
- ☐ 50 BICYCLES
- ☐ 15 WALL PUSH-UPS
- ☐ 40 RUSSIAN TWISTS

DAY 38

BREAKFAST

....
....
....
....

LUNCH

....
....
....
....

DINNER

....
....
....

SNACK

....
....
....

TODAYS WATER INTAKE

TODAYS SLEEP

SLEEP QUALITY

0   5   10

I HAVE SLEPT ..... HOURS

TODAYS FEELINGS

WORKOUT OF THE DAY

- [ ] 90 JUMPING JACKS
- [ ] 20 TRICEP DIPS
- [ ] 10 SIT-UPS
- [ ] 30 SECONDS PLANK
- [ ] 30 SQUATS
- [ ] 15 INCLINE PUSH-UPS
- [ ] 40 CRUNCHES
- [ ] 10 OBLIQUE CRUNCHES (EACH SIDE)
- [ ] 20 STANDING CALF RAISES

DAY 39

BREAKFAST

....
....
....
....

LUNCH

....
....
....
....

DINNER

....
....
....
....

SNACK

....
....
....
....

TODAYS WATER INTAKE

TODAYS SLEEP

SLEEP QUALITY

| 0 | 5 | 10 |

I HAVE SLEPT ..... HOURS

TODAYS FEELINGS

☆ ☆ ☆

WORKOUT OF THE DAY

- ☐ 100 JUMPING JACKS
- ☐ 25 VERTICAL LEG CRUNCHES
- ☐ 30 CRUNCHES
- ☐ 20 SQUATS
- ☐ 20 WALL PUSH-UPS
- ☐ 50 RUSSIAN TWISTS
- ☐ 15 SECONDS SIDE PLANK (EACH SIDE)
- ☐ 10 LUNGE SPLIT JUMPS
- ☐ 5 JUMP SQUATS
- ☐ 40 HIGH KNEES

DAY 40

BREAKFAST

....
....
....
....

LUNCH

....
....
....
....

DINNER

....
....
....
....

SNACK

....
....
....
....

TODAYS WATER INTAKE

TODAYS SLEEP

SLEEP QUALITY

| 0 | 5 | 10 |

I HAVE SLEPT ..... HOURS

TODAYS FEELINGS

WORKOUT OF THE DAY

- ☐ 60 JUMPING JACKS
- ☐ 40 CRUNCHES
- ☐ 10 SIT-UPS
- ☐ 10 TRICEP DIPS
- ☐ 20 SIDE LUNGES (EACH SIDE)
- ☐ 15 INCLINE PUSH-UPS
- ☐ 10 OBLIQUE CRUNCHES (EACH SIDE)
- ☐ 30 BUTT KICKERS
- ☐ 5 JUMP SQUATS
- ☐ 10 JACK KNIFE SIT-UPS

DAY 41

BREAKFAST

....
....
....
....

LUNCH

....
....
....
....

DINNER

....
....
....
....

SNACK

....
....
....
....

TODAYS WATER INTAKE

TODAYS SLEEP

SLEEP QUALITY

0   5   10

I HAVE SLEPT ..... HOURS

TODAYS FEELINGS

WORKOUT OF THE DAY

- ☐ 50 JUMPING JACKS
- ☐ 20 SQUATS
- ☐ 100 RUSSIAN TWISTS
- ☐ 5 KNEELING PUSH-UPS
- ☐ 1 MINUTE DOWNWARD DOG
- ☐ 15 JACK KNIFE SIT-UPS
- ☐ 10 LUNGES (EACH SIDE)
- ☐ 10 SIDE LUNGES (EACH SIDE)
- ☐ 20 INNER THIGH LIFTS (EACH SIDE)

DAY 42

BREAKFAST

....
....
....
....

LUNCH

....
....
....
....

DINNER

....
....
....
....

SNACK

....
....
....
....

TODAYS WATER INTAKE

TODAYS SLEEP

SLEEP QUALITY

0	5	10

I HAVE SLEPT ..... HOURS

TODAYS FEELINGS

WORKOUT OF THE DAY

- ☐ 45 JUMPING JACKS
- ☐ 15 SQUATS
- ☐ 5 JUMP SQUATS
- ☐ 50 RUSSIAN TWISTS
- ☐ 30 SECONDS PLANK
- ☐ 10 STANDING CALF RAISES
- ☐ 5 KNEELING PUSH-UPS
- ☐ 30 SECONDS SUPERMAN
- ☐ 10 LUNGES (EACH SIDE)
- ☐ 40 CRUNCHES

DAY 43

BREAKFAST

....
....
....
....

LUNCH

....
....
....
....

DINNER

....
....
....
....

SNACK

....
....
....
....

TODAYS WATER INTAKE

TODAYS SLEEP

SLEEP QUALITY

| 0 | 5 | 10 |

I HAVE SLEPT ..... HOURS

TODAYS FEELINGS

WORKOUT OF THE DAY

- ☐ 100 JUMPING JACKS
- ☐ 50 CRUNCHES
- ☐ 20 TRICEP DIPS
- ☐ 15 SQUATS
- ☐ 20 LUNGES (EACH SIDE)
- ☐ 70 RUSSIAN TWISTS
- ☐ 20 STANDING CALF RAISES
- ☐ 5 PUSH-UPS
- ☐ 30 SECONDS PLANK
- ☐ 10 LUNGE SPLIT JUMPS

DAY 44

BREAKFAST

....
....
....
....

LUNCH

....
....
....
....

DINNER

....
....
....
....

SNACK

....
....
....
....

TODAYS WATER INTAKE

TODAYS SLEEP

SLEEP QUALITY

0   5   10

I HAVE SLEPT ..... HOURS

TODAYS FEELINGS

WORKOUT OF THE DAY

- [ ] 80 JUMPING JACKS
- [ ] 50 VERTICAL LEG CRUNCHES
- [ ] 20 SIT-UPS
- [ ] 15 TRICEP DIPS
- [ ] 20 SQUATS
- [ ] 10 SIDE LUNGES (EACH LEG)
- [ ] 15 LEG LIFTS (EACH LEG)
- [ ] 50 BICYCLES
- [ ] 15 WALL PUSH-UPS
- [ ] 40 RUSSIAN TWISTS

DAY 45

BREAKFAST

....
....
....
....

LUNCH

....
....
....
....

DINNER

....
....
....
....

SNACK

....
....
....
....

TODAYS WATER INTAKE

TODAYS SLEEP

SLEEP QUALITY

| 0 | 5 | 10 |

I HAVE SLEPT ..... HOURS

TODAYS FEELINGS

☆ ☆ ☆

WORKOUT OF THE DAY

- ☐ 90 JUMPING JACKS
- ☐ 20 TRICEP DIPS
- ☐ 10 SIT-UPS
- ☐ 30 SECONDS PLANK
- ☐ 30 SQUATS
- ☐ 15 INCLINE PUSH-UPS
- ☐ 40 CRUNCHES
- ☐ 10 OBLIQUE CRUNCHES (EACH SIDE)
- ☐ 20 STANDING CALF RAISES

DAY 46

BREAKFAST

....
....
....
....

LUNCH

....
....
....
....

DINNER

....
....
....
....

SNACK

....
....
....
....

TODAYS WATER INTAKE

TODAYS SLEEP

SLEEP QUALITY

0	5	10

I HAVE SLEPT ..... HOURS

TODAYS FEELINGS

WORKOUT OF THE DAY

- [ ] 100 JUMPING JACKS
- [ ] 25 VERTICAL LEG CRUNCHES
- [ ] 30 CRUNCHES
- [ ] 20 SQUATS
- [ ] 20 WALL PUSH-UPS
- [ ] 50 RUSSIAN TWISTS
- [ ] 15 SECONDS SIDE PLANK (EACH SIDE)
- [ ] 10 LUNGE SPLIT JUMPS
- [ ] 5 JUMP SQUATS
- [ ] 40 HIGH KNEES

DAY 47

BREAKFAST

....
....
....

LUNCH

....
....
....
....

DINNER

....
....
....
....

SNACK

....
....
....

TODAYS WATER INTAKE

TODAYS SLEEP

SLEEP QUALITY

0   5   10

I HAVE SLEPT ..... HOURS

TODAYS FEELINGS

WORKOUT OF THE DAY

- ☐ 60 JUMPING JACKS
- ☐ 40 CRUNCHES
- ☐ 10 SIT-UPS
- ☐ 10 TRICEP DIPS
- ☐ 20 SIDE LUNGES (EACH SIDE)
- ☐ 15 INCLINE PUSH-UPS
- ☐ 10 OBLIQUE CRUNCHES (EACH SIDE)
- ☐ 30 BUTT KICKERS
- ☐ 5 JUMP SQUATS
- ☐ 10 JACK KNIFE SIT-UPS

DAY 48

BREAKFAST

....
....
....
....

LUNCH

....
....
....
....

DINNER

....
....
....
....

SNACK

....
....
....
....

TODAYS WATER INTAKE

TODAYS SLEEP

SLEEP QUALITY

| 0 | 5 | 10 |

I HAVE SLEPT ..... HOURS

TODAYS FEELINGS

☆ ☆ ☆

WORKOUT OF THE DAY

☐ 50 JUMPING JACKS

☐ 20 SQUATS

☐ 100 RUSSIAN TWISTS

☐ 5 KNEELING PUSH-UPS

☐ 1 MINUTE DOWNWARD DOG

☐ 15 JACK KNIFE SIT-UPS

☐ 10 LUNGES (EACH SIDE)

☐ 10 SIDE LUNGES (EACH SIDE)

☐ 20 INNER THIGH LIFTS (EACH SIDE)

DAY 49

BREAKFAST

....
....
....
....

LUNCH

....
....
....
....

DINNER

....
....
....
....

SNACK

....
....
....
....

TODAYS WATER INTAKE

TODAYS SLEEP

SLEEP QUALITY

0   5   10

I HAVE SLEPT ..... HOURS

TODAYS FEELINGS

WORKOUT OF THE DAY

☐ 45 JUMPING JACKS

☐ 15 SQUATS

☐ 5 JUMP SQUATS

☐ 50 RUSSIAN TWISTS

☐ 30 SECONDS PLANK

☐ 10 STANDING CALF RAISES

☐ 5 KNEELING PUSH-UPS

☐ 30 SECONDS SUPERMAN

☐ 10 LUNGES (EACH SIDE)

☐ 40 CRUNCHES

DAY 50

BREAKFAST

....

....

....

....

LUNCH

....

....

....

....

DINNER

....

....

....

....

SNACK

....

....

....

....

TODAYS WATER INTAKE

TODAYS SLEEP

SLEEP QUALITY

| 0 | 5 | 10 |

I HAVE SLEPT ..... HOURS

TODAYS FEELINGS

☆ ☆ ☆

WORKOUT OF THE DAY

- ☐ 100 JUMPING JACKS
- ☐ 50 CRUNCHES
- ☐ 20 TRICEP DIPS
- ☐ 15 SQUATS
- ☐ 20 LUNGES (EACH SIDE)
- ☐ 70 RUSSIAN TWISTS
- ☐ 20 STANDING CALF RAISES
- ☐ 5 PUSH-UPS
- ☐ 30 SECONDS PLANK
- ☐ 10 LUNGE SPLIT JUMPS

DAY 51

BREAKFAST

....

....

....

LUNCH

....

....

....

....

DINNER

....

....

....

SNACK

....

....

....

....

TODAYS WATER INTAKE

TODAYS SLEEP

SLEEP QUALITY

0   5   10

I HAVE SLEPT ..... HOURS

TODAYS FEELINGS

WORKOUT OF THE DAY

- ☐ 80 JUMPING JACKS
- ☐ 50 VERTICAL LEG CRUNCHES
- ☐ 20 SIT-UPS
- ☐ 15 TRICEP DIPS
- ☐ 20 SQUATS
- ☐ 10 SIDE LUNGES (EACH LEG)
- ☐ 15 LEG LIFTS (EACH LEG)
- ☐ 50 BICYCLES
- ☐ 15 WALL PUSH-UPS
- ☐ 40 RUSSIAN TWISTS

DAY 52

BREAKFAST

....

....

....

....

LUNCH

....

....

....

....

DINNER

....

....

....

....

SNACK

....

....

....

....

TODAYS WATER INTAKE

TODAYS SLEEP

SLEEP QUALITY

0   5   10

I HAVE SLEPT ..... HOURS

TODAYS FEELINGS

WORKOUT OF THE DAY

- [ ] 90 JUMPING JACKS
- [ ] 20 TRICEP DIPS
- [ ] 10 SIT-UPS
- [ ] 30 SECONDS PLANK
- [ ] 30 SQUATS
- [ ] 15 INCLINE PUSH-UPS
- [ ] 40 CRUNCHES
- [ ] 10 OBLIQUE CRUNCHES (EACH SIDE)
- [ ] 20 STANDING CALF RAISES

DAY 53

BREAKFAST

....

....

....

LUNCH

....

....

....

....

DINNER

....

....

....

....

SNACK

....

....

....

....

TODAYS WATER INTAKE

TODAYS SLEEP

SLEEP QUALITY

0   5   10

I HAVE SLEPT ..... HOURS

TODAYS FEELINGS

☆ ☆ ☆

WORKOUT OF THE DAY

- ☐ 100 JUMPING JACKS
- ☐ 25 VERTICAL LEG CRUNCHES
- ☐ 30 CRUNCHES
- ☐ 20 SQUATS
- ☐ 20 WALL PUSH-UPS
- ☐ 50 RUSSIAN TWISTS
- ☐ 15 SECONDS SIDE PLANK (EACH SIDE)
- ☐ 10 LUNGE SPLIT JUMPS
- ☐ 5 JUMP SQUATS
- ☐ 40 HIGH KNEES

DAY 54

BREAKFAST

....
....
....
....

LUNCH

....
....
....
....

DINNER

....
....
....
....

SNACK

....
....
....
....

TODAYS WATER INTAKE

TODAYS SLEEP

SLEEP QUALITY

| 0 | 5 | 10 |

I HAVE SLEPT ..... HOURS

TODAYS FEELINGS

WORKOUT OF THE DAY

- ☐ 60 JUMPING JACKS
- ☐ 40 CRUNCHES
- ☐ 10 SIT-UPS
- ☐ 10 TRICEP DIPS
- ☐ 20 SIDE LUNGES (EACH SIDE)
- ☐ 15 INCLINE PUSH-UPS
- ☐ 10 OBLIQUE CRUNCHES (EACH SIDE)
- ☐ 30 BUTT KICKERS
- ☐ 5 JUMP SQUATS
- ☐ 10 JACK KNIFE SIT-UPS

DAY 55

Breakfast
....
....
....
....

Lunch
....
....
....
....

Dinner
....
....
....
....

Snack
....
....
....
....

Todays Water Intake

Todays Sleep

Sleep Quality

| 0 | 5 | 10 |

I have slept ..... hours

Todays Feelings

☆ ☆ ☆

WORKOUT OF THE DAY

☐ 50 Jumping Jacks

☐ 20 Squats

☐ 100 Russian Twists

☐ 5 Kneeling Push-Ups

☐ 1 Minute Downward Dog

☐ 15 Jack Knife Sit-Ups

☐ 10 Lunges (each side)

☐ 10 Side Lunges (each side)

☐ 20 Inner Thigh Lifts (each side)

DAY 56

BREAKFAST

....
....
....
....

LUNCH

....
....
....
....

DINNER

....
....
....
....

SNACK

....
....
....
....

TODAYS WATER INTAKE

TODAYS SLEEP

SLEEP QUALITY

0   5   10

I HAVE SLEPT ..... HOURS

TODAYS FEELINGS

☆ ☆ ☆

WORKOUT OF THE DAY

- ☐ 45 JUMPING JACKS
- ☐ 15 SQUATS
- ☐ 5 JUMP SQUATS
- ☐ 50 RUSSIAN TWISTS
- ☐ 30 SECONDS PLANK
- ☐ 10 STANDING CALF RAISES
- ☐ 5 KNEELING PUSH-UPS
- ☐ 30 SECONDS SUPERMAN
- ☐ 10 LUNGES (EACH SIDE)
- ☐ 40 CRUNCHES

DAY 57

BREAKFAST

....
....
....
....

LUNCH

....
....
....
....

DINNER

....
....
....
....

SNACK

....
....
....
....

TODAYS WATER INTAKE

TODAYS SLEEP

SLEEP QUALITY

| 0 | 5 | 10 |

I HAVE SLEPT ..... HOURS

TODAYS FEELINGS

WORKOUT OF THE DAY

- ☐ 100 JUMPING JACKS
- ☐ 50 CRUNCHES
- ☐ 20 TRICEP DIPS
- ☐ 15 SQUATS
- ☐ 20 LUNGES (EACH SIDE)
- ☐ 70 RUSSIAN TWISTS
- ☐ 20 STANDING CALF RAISES
- ☐ 5 PUSH-UPS
- ☐ 30 SECONDS PLANK
- ☐ 10 LUNGE SPLIT JUMPS

DAY 58

BREAKFAST

....

....

....

....

LUNCH

....

....

....

....

DINNER

....

....

....

....

SNACK

....

....

....

....

TODAYS WATER INTAKE

TODAYS SLEEP

SLEEP QUALITY

0   5   10

I HAVE SLEPT ..... HOURS

TODAYS FEELINGS

☆ ☆ ☆

WORKOUT OF THE DAY

☐ 80 JUMPING JACKS

☐ 50 VERTICAL LEG CRUNCHES

☐ 20 SIT-UPS

☐ 15 TRICEP DIPS

☐ 20 SQUATS

☐ 10 SIDE LUNGES (EACH LEG)

☐ 15 LEG LIFTS (EACH LEG)

☐ 50 BICYCLES

☐ 15 WALL PUSH-UPS

☐ 40 RUSSIAN TWISTS

DAY 59

BREAKFAST

....
....
....
....

LUNCH

....
....
....
....

DINNER

....
....
....
....

SNACK

....
....
....

TODAYS WATER INTAKE

TODAYS SLEEP

SLEEP QUALITY

```
0          5          10
```

I HAVE SLEPT ..... HOURS

TODAYS FEELINGS

☆ ☆ ☆

WORKOUT OF THE DAY

☐ 90 JUMPING JACKS

☐ 20 TRICEP DIPS

☐ 10 SIT-UPS

☐ 30 SECONDS PLANK

☐ 30 SQUATS

☐ 15 INCLINE PUSH-UPS

☐ 40 CRUNCHES

☐ 10 OBLIQUE CRUNCHES (EACH SIDE)

☐ 20 STANDING CALF RAISES

DAY 60

BREAKFAST

....
....
....
....

LUNCH

....
....
....
....

DINNER

....
....
....
....

SNACK

....
....
....
....

TODAYS WATER INTAKE

TODAYS SLEEP

SLEEP QUALITY

| 0 | 5 | 10 |

I HAVE SLEPT ..... HOURS

TODAYS FEELINGS

WORKOUT OF THE DAY

- ☐ 100 JUMPING JACKS
- ☐ 25 VERTICAL LEG CRUNCHES
- ☐ 30 CRUNCHES
- ☐ 20 SQUATS
- ☐ 20 WALL PUSH-UPS
- ☐ 50 RUSSIAN TWISTS
- ☐ 15 SECONDS SIDE PLANK (EACH SIDE)
- ☐ 10 LUNGE SPLIT JUMPS
- ☐ 5 JUMP SQUATS
- ☐ 40 HIGH KNEES

DAY 61

Breakfast
....
....
....

Lunch
....
....
....
....

Dinner
....
....
....

Snack
....
....
....

Todays Water Intake

Todays Sleep

Sleep Quality

0   5   10

I have slept ..... hours

Todays Feelings

Workout of the day

- [ ] 60 Jumping Jacks
- [ ] 40 Crunches
- [ ] 10 Sit-Ups
- [ ] 10 Tricep Dips
- [ ] 20 Side Lunges (each side)
- [ ] 15 Incline Push-Ups
- [ ] 10 Oblique Crunches (each side)
- [ ] 30 Butt Kickers
- [ ] 5 Jump Squats
- [ ] 10 Jack Knife Sit-Ups

DAY 62

BREAKFAST

....

....

....

....

LUNCH

....

....

....

....

DINNER

....

....

....

....

SNACK

....

....

....

....

TODAYS WATER INTAKE

TODAYS SLEEP

SLEEP QUALITY

0   5   10

I HAVE SLEPT ..... HOURS

TODAYS FEELINGS

WORKOUT OF THE DAY

- ☐ 50 JUMPING JACKS
- ☐ 20 SQUATS
- ☐ 100 RUSSIAN TWISTS
- ☐ 5 KNEELING PUSH-UPS
- ☐ 1 MINUTE DOWNWARD DOG
- ☐ 15 JACK KNIFE SIT-UPS
- ☐ 10 LUNGES (EACH SIDE)
- ☐ 10 SIDE LUNGES (EACH SIDE)
- ☐ 20 INNER THIGH LIFTS (EACH SIDE)

DAY 63

BREAKFAST

....

....

....

LUNCH

....

....

....

....

DINNER

....

....

....

SNACK

....

....

....

....

TODAYS WATER INTAKE

TODAYS SLEEP

SLEEP QUALITY

0   5   10

I HAVE SLEPT ..... HOURS

TODAYS FEELINGS

WORKOUT OF THE DAY

- ☐ 45 JUMPING JACKS
- ☐ 15 SQUATS
- ☐ 5 JUMP SQUATS
- ☐ 50 RUSSIAN TWISTS
- ☐ 30 SECONDS PLANK
- ☐ 10 STANDING CALF RAISES
- ☐ 5 KNEELING PUSH-UPS
- ☐ 30 SECONDS SUPERMAN
- ☐ 10 LUNGES (EACH SIDE)
- ☐ 40 CRUNCHES

DAY 64

BREAKFAST

....
....
....
....

LUNCH

....
....
....
....

DINNER

....
....
....
....

SNACK

....
....
....
....

TODAYS WATER INTAKE

TODAYS SLEEP

SLEEP QUALITY

0	5	10

I HAVE SLEPT ..... HOURS

TODAYS FEELINGS

☆ ☆ ☆

WORKOUT OF THE DAY

- ☐ 100 JUMPING JACKS
- ☐ 50 CRUNCHES
- ☐ 20 TRICEP DIPS
- ☐ 15 SQUATS
- ☐ 20 LUNGES (EACH SIDE)
- ☐ 70 RUSSIAN TWISTS
- ☐ 20 STANDING CALF RAISES
- ☐ 5 PUSH-UPS
- ☐ 30 SECONDS PLANK
- ☐ 10 LUNGE SPLIT JUMPS

DAY 65

BREAKFAST

....

....

....

....

LUNCH

....

....

....

....

DINNER

....

....

....

....

SNACK

....

....

....

TODAYS WATER INTAKE

TODAYS SLEEP

SLEEP QUALITY

0   5   10

I HAVE SLEPT ..... HOURS

TODAYS FEELINGS

☆ ☆ ☆

WORKOUT OF THE DAY

☐ 80 JUMPING JACKS

☐ 50 VERTICAL LEG CRUNCHES

☐ 20 SIT-UPS

☐ 15 TRICEP DIPS

☐ 20 SQUATS

☐ 10 SIDE LUNGES (EACH LEG)

☐ 15 LEG LIFTS (EACH LEG)

☐ 50 BICYCLES

☐ 15 WALL PUSH-UPS

☐ 40 RUSSIAN TWISTS

DAY 66

BREAKFAST

....

....

....

....

LUNCH

....

....

....

....

DINNER

....

....

....

....

SNACK

....

....

....

....

TODAYS WATER INTAKE

TODAYS SLEEP

SLEEP QUALITY

0   5   10

I HAVE SLEPT ..... HOURS

TODAYS FEELINGS

☆ ☆ ☆

WORKOUT OF THE DAY

☐ 90 JUMPING JACKS

☐ 20 TRICEP DIPS

☐ 10 SIT-UPS

☐ 30 SECONDS PLANK

☐ 30 SQUATS

☐ 15 INCLINE PUSH-UPS

☐ 40 CRUNCHES

☐ 10 OBLIQUE CRUNCHES (EACH SIDE)

☐ 20 STANDING CALF RAISES

DAY 67

BREAKFAST

....
....
....
....

LUNCH

....
....
....
....

DINNER

....
....
....
....

SNACK

....
....
....
....

TODAYS WATER INTAKE

TODAYS SLEEP

SLEEP QUALITY

0   5   10

I HAVE SLEPT ..... HOURS

TODAYS FEELINGS

WORKOUT OF THE DAY

- ☐ 100 JUMPING JACKS
- ☐ 25 VERTICAL LEG CRUNCHES
- ☐ 30 CRUNCHES
- ☐ 20 SQUATS
- ☐ 20 WALL PUSH-UPS
- ☐ 50 RUSSIAN TWISTS
- ☐ 15 SECONDS SIDE PLANK (EACH SIDE)
- ☐ 10 LUNGE SPLIT JUMPS
- ☐ 5 JUMP SQUATS
- ☐ 40 HIGH KNEES

DAY 68

BREAKFAST

....
....
....
....

LUNCH

....
....
....
....

DINNER

....
....
....
....

SNACK

....
....
....

TODAYS WATER INTAKE

TODAYS SLEEP

SLEEP QUALITY

0   5   10

I HAVE SLEPT ..... HOURS

TODAYS FEELINGS

☆ ☆ ☆

WORKOUT OF THE DAY

- ☐ 60 JUMPING JACKS
- ☐ 40 CRUNCHES
- ☐ 10 SIT-UPS
- ☐ 10 TRICEP DIPS
- ☐ 20 SIDE LUNGES (EACH SIDE)
- ☐ 15 INCLINE PUSH-UPS
- ☐ 10 OBLIQUE CRUNCHES (EACH SIDE)
- ☐ 30 BUTT KICKERS
- ☐ 5 JUMP SQUATS
- ☐ 10 JACK KNIFE SIT-UPS

DAY 69

BREAKFAST
....
....
....
....

LUNCH
....
....
....
....

DINNER
....
....
....
....

SNACK
....
....
....
....

TODAYS WATER INTAKE

TODAYS SLEEP

SLEEP QUALITY

0   5   10

I HAVE SLEPT ..... HOURS

TODAYS FEELINGS

WORKOUT OF THE DAY

☐ 50 JUMPING JACKS

☐ 20 SQUATS

☐ 100 RUSSIAN TWISTS

☐ 5 KNEELING PUSH-UPS

☐ 1 MINUTE DOWNWARD DOG

☐ 15 JACK KNIFE SIT-UPS

☐ 10 LUNGES (EACH SIDE)

☐ 10 SIDE LUNGES (EACH SIDE)

☐ 20 INNER THIGH LIFTS (EACH SIDE)

DAY 70

BREAKFAST

....
....
....
....

LUNCH

....
....
....
....

DINNER

....
....
....

SNACK

....
....
....

TODAYS WATER INTAKE

TODAYS SLEEP

SLEEP QUALITY

0   5   10

I HAVE SLEPT ..... HOURS

TODAYS FEELINGS

☆ ☆ ☆

WORKOUT OF THE DAY

☐ 45 JUMPING JACKS

☐ 15 SQUATS

☐ 5 JUMP SQUATS

☐ 50 RUSSIAN TWISTS

☐ 30 SECONDS PLANK

☐ 10 STANDING CALF RAISES

☐ 5 KNEELING PUSH-UPS

☐ 30 SECONDS SUPERMAN

☐ 10 LUNGES (EACH SIDE)

☐ 40 CRUNCHES

DAY 71

BREAKFAST

....
....
....
....

LUNCH

....
....
....
....

DINNER

....
....
....
....

SNACK

....
....
....
....

TODAYS WATER INTAKE

TODAYS SLEEP

SLEEP QUALITY

0   5   10

I HAVE SLEPT ..... HOURS

TODAYS FEELINGS

☆ ☆ ☆

WORKOUT OF THE DAY

- ☐ 100 JUMPING JACKS
- ☐ 50 CRUNCHES
- ☐ 20 TRICEP DIPS
- ☐ 15 SQUATS
- ☐ 20 LUNGES (EACH SIDE)
- ☐ 70 RUSSIAN TWISTS
- ☐ 20 STANDING CALF RAISES
- ☐ 5 PUSH-UPS
- ☐ 30 SECONDS PLANK
- ☐ 10 LUNGE SPLIT JUMPS

DAY 72

BREAKFAST

DINNER

LUNCH

SNACK

TODAYS WATER INTAKE

TODAYS SLEEP

SLEEP QUALITY

0   5   10

I HAVE SLEPT ..... HOURS

TODAYS FEELINGS

WORKOUT OF THE DAY

- ☐ 80 JUMPING JACKS
- ☐ 50 VERTICAL LEG CRUNCHES
- ☐ 20 SIT-UPS
- ☐ 15 TRICEP DIPS
- ☐ 20 SQUATS
- ☐ 10 SIDE LUNGES (EACH LEG)
- ☐ 15 LEG LIFTS (EACH LEG)
- ☐ 50 BICYCLES
- ☐ 15 WALL PUSH-UPS
- ☐ 40 RUSSIAN TWISTS

DAY 73

BREAKFAST

....
....
....
....

LUNCH

....
....
....
....

DINNER

....
....
....
....

SNACK

....
....
....
....

TODAYS WATER INTAKE

TODAYS SLEEP

SLEEP QUALITY

0   5   10

I HAVE SLEPT ..... HOURS

TODAYS FEELINGS

WORKOUT OF THE DAY

- ☐ 90 JUMPING JACKS
- ☐ 20 TRICEP DIPS
- ☐ 10 SIT-UPS
- ☐ 30 SECONDS PLANK
- ☐ 30 SQUATS
- ☐ 15 INCLINE PUSH-UPS
- ☐ 40 CRUNCHES
- ☐ 10 OBLIQUE CRUNCHES (EACH SIDE)
- ☐ 20 STANDING CALF RAISES

DAY 74

BREAKFAST

....

....

....

....

LUNCH

....

....

....

....

DINNER

....

....

....

SNACK

....

....

....

TODAYS WATER INTAKE

TODAYS SLEEP

SLEEP QUALITY

0   5   10

I HAVE SLEPT ..... HOURS

TODAYS FEELINGS

☆ ☆ ☆

WORKOUT OF THE DAY

☐ 100 JUMPING JACKS

☐ 25 VERTICAL LEG CRUNCHES

☐ 30 CRUNCHES

☐ 20 SQUATS

☐ 20 WALL PUSH-UPS

☐ 50 RUSSIAN TWISTS

☐ 15 SECONDS SIDE PLANK (EACH SIDE)

☐ 10 LUNGE SPLIT JUMPS

☐ 5 JUMP SQUATS

☐ 40 HIGH KNEES

DAY 75

BREAKFAST

....
....
....

LUNCH

....
....
....
....

DINNER

....
....
....

SNACK

....
....
....

TODAYS WATER INTAKE

TODAYS SLEEP

SLEEP QUALITY

0   5   10

I HAVE SLEPT ..... HOURS

TODAYS FEELINGS

WORKOUT OF THE DAY

☐ 60 JUMPING JACKS

☐ 40 CRUNCHES

☐ 10 SIT-UPS

☐ 10 TRICEP DIPS

☐ 20 SIDE LUNGES (EACH SIDE)

☐ 15 INCLINE PUSH-UPS

☐ 10 OBLIQUE CRUNCHES (EACH SIDE)

☐ 30 BUTT KICKERS

☐ 5 JUMP SQUATS

☐ 10 JACK KNIFE SIT-UPS

DAY 76

BREAKFAST

....
....
....
....

LUNCH

....
....
....
....

DINNER

....
....
....
....

SNACK

....
....
....
....

TODAYS WATER INTAKE

TODAYS SLEEP

SLEEP QUALITY

| 0 | 5 | 10 |

I HAVE SLEPT ..... HOURS

TODAYS FEELINGS

WORKOUT OF THE DAY

- ☐ 50 JUMPING JACKS
- ☐ 20 SQUATS
- ☐ 100 RUSSIAN TWISTS
- ☐ 5 KNEELING PUSH-UPS
- ☐ 1 MINUTE DOWNWARD DOG
- ☐ 15 JACK KNIFE SIT-UPS
- ☐ 10 LUNGES (EACH SIDE)
- ☐ 10 SIDE LUNGES (EACH SIDE)
- ☐ 20 INNER THIGH LIFTS (EACH SIDE)

DAY 77

BREAKFAST

....
....
....

LUNCH

....
....
....
....

DINNER

....
....
....

SNACK

....
....
....

TODAYS WATER INTAKE

TODAYS SLEEP

SLEEP QUALITY

0   5   10

I HAVE SLEPT ..... HOURS

TODAYS FEELINGS

WORKOUT OF THE DAY

- [ ] 45 JUMPING JACKS
- [ ] 15 SQUATS
- [ ] 5 JUMP SQUATS
- [ ] 50 RUSSIAN TWISTS
- [ ] 30 SECONDS PLANK
- [ ] 10 STANDING CALF RAISES
- [ ] 5 KNEELING PUSH-UPS
- [ ] 30 SECONDS SUPERMAN
- [ ] 10 LUNGES (EACH SIDE)
- [ ] 40 CRUNCHES

DAY 78

BREAKFAST

....

....

....

....

LUNCH

....

....

....

....

DINNER

....

....

....

SNACK

....

....

....

....

TODAYS WATER INTAKE

TODAYS SLEEP

SLEEP QUALITY

| 0 | 5 | 10 |

I HAVE SLEPT ..... HOURS

TODAYS FEELINGS

☆ ☆ ☆

WORKOUT OF THE DAY

☐ 100 JUMPING JACKS

☐ 50 CRUNCHES

☐ 20 TRICEP DIPS

☐ 15 SQUATS

☐ 20 LUNGES (EACH SIDE)

☐ 70 RUSSIAN TWISTS

☐ 20 STANDING CALF RAISES

☐ 5 PUSH-UPS

☐ 30 SECONDS PLANK

☐ 10 LUNGE SPLIT JUMPS

DAY 79

BREAKFAST
....
....
....
....

LUNCH
....
....
....
....

DINNER
....
....
....
....

SNACK
....
....
....
....

TODAYS WATER INTAKE

TODAYS SLEEP

SLEEP QUALITY

| 0 | 5 | 10 |

I HAVE SLEPT ..... HOURS

TODAYS FEELINGS

WORKOUT OF THE DAY

- ☐ 80 JUMPING JACKS
- ☐ 50 VERTICAL LEG CRUNCHES
- ☐ 20 SIT-UPS
- ☐ 15 TRICEP DIPS
- ☐ 20 SQUATS
- ☐ 10 SIDE LUNGES (EACH LEG)
- ☐ 15 LEG LIFTS (EACH LEG)
- ☐ 50 BICYCLES
- ☐ 15 WALL PUSH-UPS
- ☐ 40 RUSSIAN TWISTS

DAY 80

BREAKFAST	DINNER
....	....
....	....
....	....
....	....
LUNCH	**SNACK**
....	....
....	....
....	....
....	....

TODAYS WATER INTAKE

TODAYS SLEEP

SLEEP QUALITY

0   5   10

I HAVE SLEPT ..... HOURS

TODAYS FEELINGS

☆ ☆ ☆

WORKOUT OF THE DAY

☐ 90 JUMPING JACKS

☐ 20 TRICEP DIPS

☐ 10 SIT-UPS

☐ 30 SECONDS PLANK

☐ 30 SQUATS

☐ 15 INCLINE PUSH-UPS

☐ 40 CRUNCHES

☐ 10 OBLIQUE CRUNCHES (EACH SIDE)

☐ 20 STANDING CALF RAISES

DAY 81

BREAKFAST

....
....
....
....

LUNCH

....
....
....
....

DINNER

....
....
....
....

SNACK

....
....
....
....

TODAYS WATER INTAKE

TODAYS SLEEP

SLEEP QUALITY

0   5   10

I HAVE SLEPT ..... HOURS

TODAYS FEELINGS

WORKOUT OF THE DAY

- ☐ 100 JUMPING JACKS
- ☐ 25 VERTICAL LEG CRUNCHES
- ☐ 30 CRUNCHES
- ☐ 20 SQUATS
- ☐ 20 WALL PUSH-UPS
- ☐ 50 RUSSIAN TWISTS
- ☐ 15 SECONDS SIDE PLANK (EACH SIDE)
- ☐ 10 LUNGE SPLIT JUMPS
- ☐ 5 JUMP SQUATS
- ☐ 40 HIGH KNEES

DAY 82

BREAKFAST

....
....
....
....

LUNCH

....
....
....
....

DINNER

....
....
....
....

SNACK

....
....
....
....

TODAYS WATER INTAKE

TODAYS SLEEP

SLEEP QUALITY

0   5   10

I HAVE SLEPT ..... HOURS

TODAYS FEELINGS

WORKOUT OF THE DAY

- [ ] 60 JUMPING JACKS
- [ ] 40 CRUNCHES
- [ ] 10 SIT-UPS
- [ ] 10 TRICEP DIPS
- [ ] 20 SIDE LUNGES (EACH SIDE)
- [ ] 15 INCLINE PUSH-UPS
- [ ] 10 OBLIQUE CRUNCHES (EACH SIDE)
- [ ] 30 BUTT KICKERS
- [ ] 5 JUMP SQUATS
- [ ] 10 JACK KNIFE SIT-UPS

DAY 83

BREAKFAST

....
....
....

LUNCH

....
....
....
....

DINNER

....
....
....
....

SNACK

....
....
....

TODAYS WATER INTAKE

TODAYS SLEEP

SLEEP QUALITY

0   5   10

I HAVE SLEPT ..... HOURS

TODAYS FEELINGS

WORKOUT OF THE DAY

☐ 50 JUMPING JACKS

☐ 20 SQUATS

☐ 100 RUSSIAN TWISTS

☐ 5 KNEELING PUSH-UPS

☐ 1 MINUTE DOWNWARD DOG

☐ 15 JACK KNIFE SIT-UPS

☐ 10 LUNGES (EACH SIDE)

☐ 10 SIDE LUNGES (EACH SIDE)

☐ 20 INNER THIGH LIFTS (EACH SIDE)

DAY 84

BREAKFAST

....
....
....
....

LUNCH

....
....
....
....

DINNER

....
....
....
....

SNACK

....
....
....
....

TODAYS WATER INTAKE

TODAYS SLEEP

SLEEP QUALITY

0   5   10

I HAVE SLEPT ..... HOURS

TODAYS FEELINGS

☆ ☆ ☆

WORKOUT OF THE DAY

☐ 45 JUMPING JACKS

☐ 15 SQUATS

☐ 5 JUMP SQUATS

☐ 50 RUSSIAN TWISTS

☐ 30 SECONDS PLANK

☐ 10 STANDING CALF RAISES

☐ 5 KNEELING PUSH–UPS

☐ 30 SECONDS SUPERMAN

☐ 10 LUNGES (EACH SIDE)

☐ 40 CRUNCHES

DAY 85

BREAKFAST

....
....
....
....

LUNCH

....
....
....
....

DINNER

....
....
....
....

SNACK

....
....
....
....

TODAYS WATER INTAKE

TODAYS SLEEP

SLEEP QUALITY

0   5   10

I HAVE SLEPT ..... HOURS

TODAYS FEELINGS

WORKOUT OF THE DAY

- [ ] 100 JUMPING JACKS
- [ ] 50 CRUNCHES
- [ ] 20 TRICEP DIPS
- [ ] 15 SQUATS
- [ ] 20 LUNGES (EACH SIDE)
- [ ] 70 RUSSIAN TWISTS
- [ ] 20 STANDING CALF RAISES
- [ ] 5 PUSH-UPS
- [ ] 30 SECONDS PLANK
- [ ] 10 LUNGE SPLIT JUMPS

DAY 86

BREAKFAST
....
....
....
....

LUNCH
....
....
....
....

DINNER
....
....
....
....

SNACK
....
....
....
....

TODAYS WATER INTAKE

TODAYS SLEEP

SLEEP QUALITY

0   5   10

I HAVE SLEPT ..... HOURS

TODAYS FEELINGS

☆ ☆ ☆

WORKOUT OF THE DAY

☐ 80 JUMPING JACKS

☐ 50 VERTICAL LEG CRUNCHES

☐ 20 SIT-UPS

☐ 15 TRICEP DIPS

☐ 20 SQUATS

☐ 10 SIDE LUNGES (EACH LEG)

☐ 15 LEG LIFTS (EACH LEG)

☐ 50 BICYCLES

☐ 15 WALL PUSH-UPS

☐ 40 RUSSIAN TWISTS

DAY 87

BREAKFAST

....
....
....
....

LUNCH

....
....
....
....

DINNER

....
....
....
....

SNACK

....
....
....
....

TODAYS WATER INTAKE

TODAYS SLEEP

SLEEP QUALITY

0   5   10

I HAVE SLEPT ..... HOURS

TODAYS FEELINGS

☆ ☆ ☆

WORKOUT OF THE DAY

- ☐ 90 JUMPING JACKS
- ☐ 20 TRICEP DIPS
- ☐ 10 SIT-UPS
- ☐ 30 SECONDS PLANK
- ☐ 30 SQUATS
- ☐ 15 INCLINE PUSH-UPS
- ☐ 40 CRUNCHES
- ☐ 10 OBLIQUE CRUNCHES (EACH SIDE)
- ☐ 20 STANDING CALF RAISES

DAY 88

BREAKFAST

....
....
....
....

LUNCH

....
....
....
....

DINNER

....
....
....
....

SNACK

....
....
....

TODAYS WATER INTAKE

TODAYS SLEEP

SLEEP QUALITY

0   5   10

I HAVE SLEPT ..... HOURS

TODAYS FEELINGS

WORKOUT OF THE DAY

- ☐ 100 JUMPING JACKS
- ☐ 25 VERTICAL LEG CRUNCHES
- ☐ 30 CRUNCHES
- ☐ 20 SQUATS
- ☐ 20 WALL PUSH-UPS
- ☐ 50 RUSSIAN TWISTS
- ☐ 15 SECONDS SIDE PLANK (EACH SIDE)
- ☐ 10 LUNGE SPLIT JUMPS
- ☐ 5 JUMP SQUATS
- ☐ 40 HIGH KNEES

DAY 89

BREAKFAST
....
....
....

LUNCH
....
....
....
....

DINNER
....
....
....
....

SNACK
....
....
....

TODAYS WATER INTAKE

TODAYS SLEEP

SLEEP QUALITY

0   5   10

I HAVE SLEPT ..... HOURS

TODAYS FEELINGS

WORKOUT OF THE DAY

- [ ] 60 JUMPING JACKS
- [ ] 40 CRUNCHES
- [ ] 10 SIT-UPS
- [ ] 10 TRICEP DIPS
- [ ] 20 SIDE LUNGES (EACH SIDE)
- [ ] 15 INCLINE PUSH-UPS
- [ ] 10 OBLIQUE CRUNCHES (EACH SIDE)
- [ ] 30 BUTT KICKERS
- [ ] 5 JUMP SQUATS
- [ ] 10 JACK KNIFE SIT-UPS

DAY 90

BREAKFAST

....
....
....

LUNCH

....
....
....
....

DINNER

....
....
....
....

SNACK

....
....
....
....

TODAYS WATER INTAKE

TODAYS SLEEP

SLEEP QUALITY

0   5   10

I HAVE SLEPT ..... HOURS

TODAYS FEELINGS

WORKOUT OF THE DAY

- [ ] 50 JUMPING JACKS
- [ ] 20 SQUATS
- [ ] 100 RUSSIAN TWISTS
- [ ] 5 KNEELING PUSH-UPS
- [ ] 1 MINUTE DOWNWARD DOG
- [ ] 15 JACK KNIFE SIT-UPS
- [ ] 10 LUNGES (EACH SIDE)
- [ ] 10 SIDE LUNGES (EACH SIDE)
- [ ] 20 INNER THIGH LIFTS (EACH SIDE)

www.ingramcontent.com/pod-product-compliance
Lightning Source LLC
Chambersburg PA
CBHW051356280526
45784CB00007B/2988